FLEXITARIAN DIET COOKBOOK

100 Delicious Beginners Recipes, Smoothies' Snacks And Meal Plan

Embrace A Balanced Eating Style That Incorporates More Plant-Based Foods For Long-Term Health

Dr. Belinda Bianca

Table of Contents

CHAPTER ONE

Introduction

Flexitarian diets, which prioritize plant-based meals while allowing for the occasional intake of meat and other animal products, have grown in favor in recent years due to their various health and environmental advantages.

In this article, we will look at the benefits of a flexitarian diet, go over plant-based foods, provide advice for switching to a flexitarian lifestyle, and explain the necessity of macronutrient balance within this dietary strategy.

10 Advantages Of A Flexitarian Diet

1. Flexitarians eat more fruits, vegetables, whole grains, and legumes, which are high in critical nutrients, antioxidants, and fiber. This eating pattern is linked to a lower risk of chronic

illnesses including heart disease, diabetes, and some malignancies.

2. Weight Management: Flexitarian diets are frequently lower in calories and saturated fats than standard meat-heavy meals, making them ideal for weight reduction and management objectives.

3. Environmental Sustainability: Plant-based meals have a lighter environmental footprint than animal goods because they utilize fewer resources such as water and land and emit fewer greenhouse gases. Flexitarians help the environment by lowering their meat intake.

4. Economic Savings: Plant-based proteins such as beans, lentils, and tofu are often less expensive than meat, making a flexitarian diet a viable choice for many people and families.

5. Digestive Health: Plant-based meals' high fiber content supports good digestion and may lower the

risk of constipation, diverticulosis, and other gastrointestinal problems.

6. Flexitarians are less likely to get foodborne illnesses because they reduce their dependence on animal products.

7. Ethical Considerations: Flexitarianism enables people to connect their food choices with their ethical ideals by decreasing animal suffering and encouraging more humane and sustainable agricultural methods.

8. Improved Energy Levels: Plant-based meals are high in vitamins, minerals, and phytonutrients, which may boost overall energy levels and encourage feelings of vitality and well-being.

9. Diverse Culinary Exploration: Following a flexitarian diet enables people to explore a broad range of plant-based foods and cooking methods, resulting in increased culinary innovation and pleasure.

10. lifespan and Disease Prevention: Research indicates that plant-based diets, especially flexitarianism, are related to increased lifespan and a lower risk of death from all causes.

Understanding Plant-Based Foods

Plant-based foods include a diverse range of fruits and vegetables, whole grains, legumes, nuts, seeds, and plant-derived goods. These foods provide critical elements such as vitamins, minerals, antioxidants, and phytonutrients, which are good for your general health and well-being. A plant-based diet consists of the following key components:

Flexitarian diets rely heavily on fruits and vegetables for their high vitamin, mineral, and fiber content. To increase nutritional absorption, choose a range of colors and varieties.

• Whole grains such as quinoa, brown rice, oats, and whole wheat include complex carbs, fiber, and minerals needed for sustained energy and overall health.

• Legumes such as beans, lentils, and chickpeas include high levels of plant-based protein, fiber, iron, and minerals. They may be a healthy substitute for meat in a variety of recipes.

• Nuts and seeds include beneficial lipids, protein, vitamins, and minerals. Incorporating them into meals and snacks enhances taste, texture, and nutrition.

• Plant-Derived Protein Sources: Tofu, tempeh, seitan, and other plant-based proteins are versatile and may replace meat in a flexitarian diet.

Getting Started: Moving To A Flexitarian Lifestyle

Transitioning to a flexitarian lifestyle requires incremental adjustments in food habits and mentality. Here are some practical strategies to help you transition:

• Begin slowly by increasing plant-based meals and decreasing meat intake. Begin with one or two vegetarian days each week, gradually increasing as you feel more comfortable.

• Prioritize healthy, minimally processed plant foods, including fruits, vegetables, whole grains, and legumes. These foods are nutrition-packed and promote general wellness.

• Try new plant-based dishes from cookbooks, internet, and blogs. Experiment with various ingredients and cooking techniques to get new tastes and sensations.

• Plan and prepare meals ahead of time for a balanced and enjoyable diet. Batch cooking and meal preparation may save time and help you keep to your nutritional objectives throughout the week.

• Seek assistance from online forums, culinary courses, or friends and family who have similar nutritional objectives. Having a support network might help you stay encouraged and motivated.

• Flexibility is essential for maintaining a flexitarian lifestyle. Allow yourself to sometimes consume animal products without shame or judgment.

Balancing Macronutrients In A Flexitarian Diet

A balanced macronutrient intake—carbohydrates, proteins, and fats—is critical for maximum health and well-being on a flexitarian diet. Below are some suggestions for balancing macronutrients:

• Eat complex carbs such as whole grains, fruits, vegetables, and legumes. These meals give long-lasting energy and necessary nutrients.

• Incorporate plant-based protein sources such as beans, lentils, tofu, tempeh, nuts, and seeds into your meals to meet necessary amino acid requirements.

• Consume healthy fats like avocados, nuts, seeds, olives, and plant-based oils. Limit the amount of saturated and trans fats in processed and fried meals, as well as animal products.

• Fiber: Eat plenty of fruits, vegetables, whole grains, and legumes. Fiber improves digestive health, regulates blood sugar levels, and increases feelings of fullness.

• Ensure adequate consumption of micronutrients including calcium, iron, vitamin B12, and omega-3 fatty acids in plant-based diets by supplementation or strategic food choices.

Individuals may reap the multiple health advantages of a flexitarian diet by emphasizing nutrient-dense plant foods, experimenting with new dishes, and being flexible in their dietary choices.

CHAPTER TWO

100 Delicious Meals And Preparation Procedures

Preparing meals from home provides a wide range of tastes, textures, and enjoyment that prepackaged foods cannot equal. We've produced a list of 100 delectable dishes, complete with preparation instructions, to inspire your culinary adventures.

1. Spaghetti Carbonara

• Cook spaghetti according to package directions.

• In a pan, cook the pancetta until crispy.

• Mix eggs, Parmesan cheese, and black pepper.

• Combine cooked pasta, egg mixture, and pancetta.

2. Chicken Tikka Masala

• Marinate chicken with yogurt, spices, and lemon juice.

• Grill or bake marinated chicken until done.

• Create a sauce using tomatoes, cream, and spices.

• Simmer cooked chicken in sauce until flavors combine.

3. Beef Wellington

• Brown beef fillet.

• Spread mustard on the fillet and wrap in puff pastry.

• Bake until crust is golden brown and meat is cooked to your preferred doneness.

4. Vegetable Stir-Fry.

• Chop several veggies, including bell peppers, broccoli, and carrots.

• Stir-fry veggies in a heated skillet with garlic and ginger.

• Season with soy sauce and other ingredients to taste.

5. Margherita Pizza

To make pizza dough, combine flour, yeast, water, and salt.

• Roll out dough and top with tomato sauce, mozzarella, and basil.

• Bake in a hot oven until the crust is crispy and the cheese is bubbling.

6. Beef Stroganoff

• Brown sliced beef with onions and mushrooms.

• Combine beef broth, sour cream, and mustard in the pan.

• Simmer until the sauce thickens and the flavors combine.

• Serve with cooked egg noodles.

7. Sushi rolls

• Cook sushi rice according to package directions.

• Fill nori sheets with cucumber, avocado, and raw fish. Spread rice on top.

• Roll firmly and cut into pieces.

8. Chicken Parmesan

• Bread chicken breasts using flour, egg, and breadcrumbs.

• Cook breaded chicken till golden brown.

• Top with marinara and mozzarella cheese.

• Bake until cheese melts and bubbles.

9. Pad Thai

• Soak rice noodles in boiling water to soften.

• Sauté shrimp, tofu, or chicken in garlic and onions.

• Combine noodles, bean sprouts, and a sauce with tamarind, fish sauce, and sugar.

• Cook noodles until fully cooked and covered with sauce.

10. Beef Tacos

• Season ground beef with taco seasoning and sauté until brown.

• Heat taco shells in the oven.

• Fill tortilla shells with meat, lettuce, tomato, cheese, and salsa.

11. Roast Chicken

• Coat chicken with olive oil, salt, pepper, and herbs.

• Oven roast until golden brown and fully done.

• Let rest before carving.

12. Lasagna

• Cook lasagna noodles to al dente.

• Combine noodles, ricotta cheese, marinara sauce, and mozzarella cheese.

• Bake in layers until bubbling and golden.

13. Shrimp Scampi.

• Sauté shrimp with garlic, butter, and white wine.

• Combine cooked spaghetti and chopped parsley.

• Garnish with a squeeze of lemon.

14. Beef Bourguignon

• Brown beef pieces.

• Sauté onions, carrots, and mushrooms in a single pan.

• Return meat to the pan with red wine and beef broth.

• Simmer until the steak is cooked and the sauce thickens.

15. Chicken Caesar Salad

• Grill or bake chicken breasts until done.

• Combine chopped romaine lettuce and Caesar dressing.

• Add sliced chicken, croutons, and grated Parmesan cheese.

16. Ratatouille

• Sauté the onions, bell peppers, zucchini, and eggplant until soft.

• Combine tomato, garlic, and herbs.

• Simmer veggies until fully cooked.

17. Beef and Broccoli

• Stir fried beef pieces with garlic and ginger.

• Stir-fry broccoli florets until soft and crisp.

• Season with soy sauce and other ingredients to taste.

18. Chicken Alfredo

• Cook the fettuccine pasta until al dente.

• Sauté chicken strips till cooked thoroughly.

• Combine cooked pasta, Alfredo sauce, and chicken.

• Garnish with grated Parmesan cheese.

19. Miso Soup

• Prepare dashi broth with kombu and bonito flakes.

• Add miso paste and stir until dissolved.

• Combine tofu, seaweed, and green onion.

• Simmer until flavors mingle.

20. Shepherd's pie.

• Brown ground beef with onions and garlic.

• Place the meat mixture in a baking dish.

• Cover with mashed potatoes and bake until golden brown.

21. Fish and chips.

• Coat fish fillets with beer batter.

• Fry until crispy and golden brown.

• Serve with thick-cut fries and tartar sauce.

22. Mushroom risotto

• Sauté mushrooms, garlic, and shallots.

• Stir in Arborio rice to coat with oil.

• Gradually add chicken or veggie broth and stir frequently.

• Combine the Parmesan cheese and butter until creamy.

23. Chicken Satay

• Marinate chicken strips in coconut milk, soy sauce, and spices.

• Grill chicken on skewers until well done.

• Complement with peanut sauce and cucumber salad.

24. Quiche Lorraine

• Blind bake pie crust.

• Sauté bacon and onions until browned.

• Combine eggs, cream, and cheese.

• Pour the egg mixture into the crust and bake until firm.

25. Beef Chili

• Brown ground beef with onions and garlic.

• Combine tomatoes, beans, chili powder, and other spices.

• Simmer until the flavors combine and the chili thickens.

26. Chicken Curry

• Sauté chicken with onion, garlic, and curry paste.

• Simmer chicken in coconut milk until fully done.

• Garnish with cilantro and serve over rice.

27. Tuna Nicoise Salad.

• Place mixed greens on a platter.

• Garnish with canned tuna, boiled potatoes, green beans, hard-boiled eggs, cherry tomatoes, and olives.

• Drizzle with vinaigrette dressing.

28. Steak Frites.

• Grill or pan-sear beef to the desired doneness.

• Pair with crispy French fries and a side salad.

29. Chicken Fajitas

• Sauté chicken strips, bell peppers, and onions.

• Serve with warm tortillas, salsa, guacamole, and sour cream.

30. Lobster Bisque.

• Sauté lobster shells, onions, carrots, and celery.

• Add broth and boil until flavors combine.

• Strain out solids and mix until smooth.

• Add cream and season to taste.

31. Beef Kebabs

• Marinate beef cubes with olive oil, garlic, and seasonings.

• Skewer beef with veggies such as bell peppers, onions, and cherry tomatoes.

• Grill meat till the desired doneness.

32. Chicken Noodle Soup

• Sauté onions, carrots, and celery until tender.

• Bring chicken broth to a boil.

• Combine cooked chicken, noodles, and seasonings.

• Simmer until flavors mingle.

33. Falafel Wraps

• Combine chickpeas, herbs, and spices in a food processor.

• Form the mixture into balls and cook until golden brown.

• Prepare a wrap with lettuce, tomato, cucumber, and tahini sauce.

34. Eggs Benedict.

• Poach eggs until whites set but yolks remain liquid.

• Toast English muffins and top with Canadian bacon or smoked salmon.

• Top with poached eggs and pour with hollandaise sauce.

35. Beef Gyros.

• Marinate thinly sliced beef with yogurt, lemon juice, and seasonings.

• Grill meat until cooked through.

• Combine pita bread with tzatziki sauce, lettuce, tomato, and onion.

36. Chicken Piccata

• Coat chicken cutlets with flour and spices.

• Sauté chicken with butter and olive oil until golden brown.

• Deglaze the pan with white wine and lemon juice.

• Simmer until sauce thickens and serve with prepared pasta.

37. Spanakopita

• Sauté spinach, garlic, and onions until wilted.

• Mix in feta cheese and herbs.

• Place spinach mixture over phyllo dough and brush with butter.

• Bake until golden brown and crunchy.

38. Chicken Shawarma

• Marinate chicken thighs with yogurt, garlic, and spices.

• Grill or roast until cooked thoroughly.

• Fill pita bread with tahini sauce, lettuce, tomato, and cucumber.

39. Beef empanadas.

• Brown ground beef with onions, garlic, and seasonings.

• Fill the empanada dough with meat mixture.

• Seal and bake until golden and crispy.

40. Chicken Teriyaki

• Marinate chicken with soy sauce, ginger, and garlic.

• Grill or pan-sear until cooked thoroughly.

• Serve with teriyaki sauce, rice, and veggies.

41. Caprese Salad

• Place sliced tomatoes, fresh mozzarella, and basil leaves on a platter.

• Drizzle balsamic glaze and olive oil.

• Season with salt and pepper.

42. Beef Pho

• Prepare broth by boiling beef bones with aromatic ingredients.

• Cook rice noodles according to package directions.

• Combine noodles in broth with thinly sliced beef, bean sprouts, lime wedges, and herbs.

43. Chicken enchiladas

• Fill tortillas with shredded chicken, cheese, and enchilada sauce.

- Roll up and put in baking dish.

- Top with more sauce and cheese.

- Bake until cheese melts and bubbles.

44. Greek Salad

- Combine diced cucumbers, tomatoes, red onions, olives, and feta cheese in a bowl.

- Drizzle with olive oil, lemon juice, and oregano.

- Season with salt and pepper.

45. Beef Bulgogi

- Marinate thinly sliced beef with soy sauce, sugar, garlic, and sesame oil.

- Grill or pan-sear until caramelized and cooked thoroughly.

- Serve with rice and kimchi.

46. Chicken Caesar Wraps

• Combine chopped romaine lettuce and Caesar dressing.

• Fill wraps with lettuce, grilled chicken, croutons, and Parmesan cheese.

47. Beef Rendang

• Combine spices including lemongrass, galangal, and chili peppers.

• Sauté the spice paste until aromatic.

• Simmer the meat and coconut milk until tender and the sauce thickens.

48. Chicken tenders

• Coat chicken strips with flour, egg, and breadcrumbs.

• Fry till golden brown and crispy.

• Pair with dipping sauces like honey mustard or barbecue.

49. Margarita Pasta

• Cook pasta until al dente.

• Sauté cherry tomatoes with garlic and red pepper flakes.

• Combine cooked pasta, tomatoes, fresh basil, and Parmesan cheese.

50. Beef tamales

• For masa dough, combine masa harina, lard, and broth.

• Fill corn husks with masa dough and shredded meat.

• Steam until cooked thoroughly.

51. Chicken Quesadillas.

• Fill tortillas with shredded chicken, cheese, and salsa.

• Fold in half and fry in a pan until crispy and cheese melted.

• Serve with sour cream and guacamole.

52. Ratatouille

• Sauté the onions, bell peppers, zucchini, and eggplant until soft.

• Combine tomato, garlic, and herbs.

• Simmer veggies until fully cooked.

53. Beef and Broccoli

• Stir fried beef pieces with garlic and ginger.

• Stir-fry broccoli florets until soft and crisp.

• Season with soy sauce and other ingredients to taste.

54. Chicken Alfredo

• Cook the fettuccine pasta until al dente.

• Sauté chicken strips till cooked thoroughly.

• Combine cooked pasta, Alfredo sauce, and chicken.

• Garnish with grated Parmesan cheese.

55. Miso Soup

• Prepare dashi broth with kombu and bonito flakes.

• Add miso paste and stir until dissolved.

• Combine tofu, seaweed, and green onion.

• Simmer until flavors mingle.

56. Shepherd's pie.

• Brown ground beef with onions and garlic.

• Place the meat mixture in a baking dish.

• Cover with mashed potatoes and bake until golden brown.

57. Fish and chips.

• Coat fish fillets with beer batter.

• Fry until crispy and golden brown.

• Serve with thick-cut fries and tartar sauce.

58. Mushroom risotto

• Sauté mushrooms, garlic, and shallots.

• Stir in Arborio rice to coat with oil.

• Gradually add chicken or veggie broth and stir frequently.

• Combine the Parmesan cheese and butter until creamy.

59. Chicken Satay

• Marinate chicken strips in coconut milk, soy sauce, and spices.

• Grill chicken on skewers until well done.

• Complement with peanut sauce and cucumber salad.

60. Quiche Lorraine

• Blind bake pie crust.

• Sauté bacon and onions until browned.

• Combine eggs, cream, and cheese.

• Pour the egg mixture into the crust and bake until firm.

61. Beef Chili

• Brown ground beef with onions and garlic.

• Combine tomatoes, beans, chili powder, and other spices.

• Simmer until the flavors combine and the chili thickens.

62. Chicken Curry

- Sauté chicken with onion, garlic, and curry paste.

- Simmer chicken in coconut milk until fully done.

- Garnish with cilantro and serve over rice.

63. Tuna Nicoise Salad.

- Place mixed greens on a platter.

- Garnish with canned tuna, boiled potatoes, green beans, hard-boiled eggs, cherry tomatoes, and olives.

- Drizzle with vinaigrette dressing.

64. Steak Frites.

- Grill or pan-sear beef to the desired doneness.

- Pair with crispy French fries and a side salad.

65. Chicken Fajitas

- Sauté chicken strips, bell peppers, and onions.

• Serve with warm tortillas, salsa, guacamole, and sour cream.

66. Lobster Bisque.

• Sauté lobster shells, onions, carrots, and celery.

• Add broth and boil until flavors combine.

• Strain out solids and mix until smooth.

• Add cream and season to taste.

67. Beef Kebabs

• Marinate beef cubes with olive oil, garlic, and seasonings.

• Skewer beef with veggies such as bell peppers, onions, and cherry tomatoes.

• Grill meat till the desired doneness.

68. Chicken Noodle Soup

• Sauté onions, carrots, and celery until tender.

• Bring chicken broth to a boil.

• Combine cooked chicken, noodles, and seasonings.

• Simmer until flavors mingle.

69. Falafel Wraps

• Combine chickpeas, herbs, and spices in a food processor.

• Form the mixture into balls and cook until golden brown.

• Prepare a wrap with lettuce, tomato, cucumber, and tahini sauce.

70. Eggs Benedict.

• Poach eggs until whites set but yolks remain liquid.

• Toast English muffins and top with Canadian bacon or smoked salmon.

• Top with poached eggs and pour with hollandaise sauce.

71. Beef Gyros.

• Marinate thinly sliced beef with yogurt, lemon juice, and seasonings.

• Grill meat until cooked through.

• Combine pita bread with tzatziki sauce, lettuce, tomato, and onion.

72. Chicken Piccata

• Coat chicken cutlets with flour and spices.

• Sauté chicken with butter and olive oil until golden brown.

• Deglaze the pan with white wine and lemon juice.

• Simmer until sauce thickens and serve with prepared pasta.

73. Spanakopita

• Sauté spinach, garlic, and onions until wilted.

• Mix in feta cheese and herbs.

• Place spinach mixture over phyllo dough and brush with butter.

• Bake until golden brown and crunchy.

74. Chicken Shawarma

• Marinate chicken thighs with yogurt, garlic, and spices.

• Grill or roast until cooked thoroughly.

• Fill pita bread with tahini sauce, lettuce, tomato, and cucumber.

75. Beef empanadas.

• Brown ground beef with onions, garlic, and seasonings.

• Fill the empanada dough with meat mixture.

• Seal and bake until golden and crispy.

76. Chicken Teriyaki

• Marinate chicken with soy sauce, ginger, and garlic.

• Grill or pan-sear until cooked thoroughly.

• Serve with teriyaki sauce, rice, and veggies.

77. Caprese Salad

• Place sliced tomatoes, fresh mozzarella, and basil leaves on a platter.

• Drizzle balsamic glaze and olive oil

• Season with salt and pepper.

78. Beef Pho

• Prepare broth by boiling beef bones with aromatic ingredients.

• Cook rice noodles according to package directions.

• Combine noodles in broth with thinly sliced beef, bean sprouts, lime wedges, and herbs.

79. Chicken enchiladas

• Fill tortillas with shredded chicken, cheese, and enchilada sauce.

• Roll up and put in baking dish.

• Top with more sauce and cheese.

• Bake until cheese melts and bubbles.

80. Greek Salad

• Combine diced cucumbers, tomatoes, red onions, olives, and feta cheese in a bowl.

• Drizzle with olive oil, lemon juice, and oregano.

• Season with salt and pepper.

81. Beef Bulgogi

• Marinate thinly sliced beef with soy sauce, sugar, garlic, and sesame oil.

• Grill or pan-sear until caramelized and cooked thoroughly.

• Serve with rice and kimchi.

82. Chicken Caesar Wraps

• Combine chopped romaine lettuce and Caesar dressing.

• Fill wraps with lettuce, grilled chicken, croutons, and Parmesan cheese.

83. Beef Rendang

• Combine spices including lemongrass, galangal, and chili peppers.

• Sauté the spice paste until aromatic.

• Simmer the meat and coconut milk until tender and the sauce thickens.

84. Chicken tenders

• Coat chicken strips with flour, egg, and breadcrumbs.

• Fry till golden brown and crispy.

• Pair with dipping sauces like honey mustard or barbecue.

85. Margarita Pasta

• Cook pasta until al dente.

• Sauté cherry tomatoes with garlic and red pepper flakes.

• Combine cooked pasta, tomatoes, fresh basil, and Parmesan cheese.

86. Beef tamales

• For masa dough, combine masa harina, lard, and broth.

• Fill corn husks with masa dough and shredded meat.

• Steam until cooked thoroughly.

87. Chicken Quesadillas.

• Fill tortillas with shredded chicken, cheese, and salsa.

• Fold in half and fry in a pan until crispy and cheese melted.

• Serve with sour cream and guacamole.

88. Ratatouille

• Sauté the onions, bell peppers, zucchini, and eggplant until soft.

• Combine tomato, garlic, and herbs.

• Simmer veggies until fully cooked.

89. Beef and Broccoli

• Stir fried beef pieces with garlic and ginger.

• Stir-fry broccoli florets until soft and crisp.

• Season with soy sauce and other ingredients to taste.

90. Chicken Alfredo

• Cook the fettuccine pasta until al dente.

• Sauté chicken strips till cooked thoroughly.

• Combine cooked pasta, Alfredo sauce, and chicken.

• Garnish with grated Parmesan cheese.

91. Miso Soup

• Prepare dashi broth with kombu and bonito flakes.

• Add miso paste and stir until dissolved.

• Combine tofu, seaweed, and green onion.

• Simmer until flavors mingle.

92. Shepherd's pie.

• Brown ground beef with onions and garlic.

• Place the meat mixture in a baking dish.

• Cover with mashed potatoes and bake until golden brown.

93. Fish and chips.

• Coat fish fillets with beer batter.

• Fry until crispy and golden brown.

• Serve with thick-cut fries and tartar sauce.

94. Mushroom risotto

• Sauté mushrooms, garlic, and shallots.

• Stir in Arborio rice to coat with oil.

- Gradually add chicken or veggie broth and stir frequently.

- Combine the Parmesan cheese and butter until creamy.

95. Chicken Satay

- Marinate chicken strips in coconut milk, soy sauce, and spices.

- Grill chicken on skewers until well done.

- Complement with peanut sauce and cucumber salad.

96. Quiche Lorraine

- Blind bake pie crust.

- Sauté bacon and onions until browned.

- Combine eggs, cream, and cheese.

• Pour the egg mixture into the crust and bake until firm.

97. Beef Chili

• Brown ground beef with onions and garlic.

• Combine tomatoes, beans, chili powder, and other spices.

• Simmer until the flavors combine and the chili thickens.

98. Chicken Curry

• Sauté chicken with onion, garlic, and curry paste.

• Simmer chicken in coconut milk until fully done.

• Garnish with cilantro and serve over rice.

99. Tuna Nicoise Salad.

• Place mixed greens on a platter.

• Garnish with canned tuna, boiled potatoes, green beans, hard-boiled eggs, cherry tomatoes, and olives.

• Drizzle with vinaigrette dressing.

100. Steak Frites.

• Grill or pan-sear beef to the desired doneness.

• Pair with crispy French fries and a side salad.

These 100 delectable dishes span a variety of cultures and preparation styles, giving unlimited inspiration for your culinary adventures. Whether you're wanting comfort cuisine, exotic tastes, or anything in between, this list has something for everyone's taste. Enjoy studying these recipes and treating your taste senses to handmade bliss.

CHAPTER THREE

Essential Kitchen Tools For Flexitarian Cooking

1. Chef's Knife: A sharp, strong chef's knife is essential for easily slicing vegetables, fruits, and meats.

2. Cutting Board: Purchase a sturdy cutting board to safeguard your surfaces while preparing ingredients.

3. Vegetable Peeler: A dependable peeler can help you quickly peel vegetables and fruits.

4. Cast iron skillets are versatile and sturdy, making them ideal for searing vegetables, meats, and even baking.

5. A blender or food processor is essential for producing smoothies, sauces, and purees, and it increases the diversity of your cuisine.

6. A quality baking sheet is a kitchen necessity that may be used to roast vegetables, bake biscuits, or reheat leftovers.

7. Instant-Read Thermometer: Use an instant-read thermometer to ensure that your meats are always perfectly done.

8. A non-stick pan is crucial for frying eggs, pancakes, and other delicate meals without worrying about them sticking.

9. With a grater or microplane, you can easily grate cheese, zest citrus, and grate spices.

10. culinary shears are flexible tools that may be used for a variety of culinary activities, including snipping herbs and cutting chicken.

5-Day Meal Plan For Success

• On Day 1, start the week with a robust veggie stir-fry over quinoa or brown rice.

• On Day 2, prepare a nutritious salad with mixed greens, roasted veggies, chickpeas, and a delicious vinaigrette.

• On Day 3, have a bowl of vegetable soup with whole-grain bread or crackers.

• Day 4: Enjoy a colorful Buddha bowl with roasted sweet potatoes, black beans, avocado, and salsa.

• Day 5: Enjoy a handmade pizza with veggies and cheese.

Stock Your Pantry With Flexitarian Staples

• Store canned and dry legumes such as black beans, chickpeas, and lentils for protein-rich meals.

• Stock up on nutritious grains like quinoa, brown rice, oats, and pasta to make healthful recipes.

• Nuts and seeds: Include almonds, walnuts, chia seeds, and flaxseeds in your meals for added crunch and nutrients.

• Canned tomatoes are a versatile pantry staple, making them ideal for sauces, soups, and stews.

• Add flavor to your recipes with spices and herbs like garlic powder, cumin, paprika, and basil.

Exploring Flavor Profiles In Flexitarian Cuisine

• Use Asian-inspired flavors such as soy sauce, ginger, garlic, and sesame oil to make flavorful stir-fries and noodles.

• Incorporate Mediterranean flavors like olive oil, lemon, oregano, and feta cheese in salads and grain bowls.

• For tasty Mexican cuisine, use chili powder, cumin, cilantro, and lime in tacos, burritos, and bowls.

Quick And Easy Flexitarian Breakfasts

1. Avocado bread: Top whole-grain bread with mashed avocado, cherry tomatoes, and a pinch of salt & pepper.

2. Smoothie Bowl: Combine frozen fruits, spinach, yogurt, and a splash of milk; top with granola and sliced bananas.

3. Greek Yogurt Parfait: For a protein-rich breakfast, combine Greek yogurt, berries, honey, and oats.

Healthy Flexitarian Lunch Ideas

1. Quinoa Salad: Toss cooked quinoa with roasted veggies, chickpeas, feta cheese, and lemon vinaigrette.

2. Fill a whole-grain wrap with hummus, mixed greens, shredded carrots, cucumber, and avocado.

3. Stuffed Sweet Potatoes: Bake sweet potatoes and fill them with black beans, salsa, avocado, and Greek yogurt.

Satisfying Flexitarian Dinners

1. Vegetable Stir-Fry: Sauté a variety of colorful veggies with tofu or tempeh in a tasty sauce before serving over brown rice or noodles.

2. Chickpea Curry: Simmer chickpeas in a spicy tomato-coconut sauce, then serve over naan bread or rice.

3. Mushroom Risotto: Make a creamy risotto with mushrooms, onions, garlic, and vegetable broth. Top with Parmesan cheese and parsley.

CHAPTER FOUR

Creative Flexitarian Snacks & Appetizers

Flexitarian snacks and appetizers allow you to explore a wide variety of plant-based components, delivering both nutrition and taste. Fruits, vegetables, whole grains, nuts, and seeds may all be combined to make snacks that are not only tasty but also high in nutrients. Examples include:

• Stuffed Mini Peppers: Add quinoa, black beans, corn, and salsa for a colorful and protein-rich snack.

• Top baked sweet potato rounds with avocado, cherry tomatoes, and feta cheese for a flavorful and healthy appetizer.

• Try several types of homemade hummus, including roasted red pepper, spinach, artichoke, or spicy avocado. Serve with healthy grain crackers or vegetable sticks.

Adding Smoothies To Your Flexitarian Diet

Smoothies provide a practical and varied option to increase nutrient consumption while following a flexitarian diet. Smoothies, which are made by combining fruits, vegetables, protein sources, and healthy fats, maybe a delicious snack or meal substitute. Key factors include:

• For a balanced meal, include a variety of fruits (e.g., berries, bananas, or mango), leafy greens (e.g., spinach or kale), protein sources (e.g., tofu, Greek yogurt, plant-based protein powder), and healthy fats (e.g., nut butter, avocado).

• For hydration, use coconut water, almond milk, or simple water. Add flavor with fresh ginger, citrus zest, or herbs such as mint or basil.

• To get a creamier texture, adjust the quantity of liquid and add ingredients such as oats, chia seeds, or frozen bananas.

Nutrient-Dense Flexitarian Desserts

Desserts may be both decadent and nutritious on a flexitarian diet, including healthy ingredients while satisfying sweet cravings. Desserts may complement a healthy diet by concentrating on nutritional density and portion sizes. Examples include:

• For a fiber-rich dessert, mix chia seeds, almond milk, vanilla essence, and maple syrup. Refrigerate until thickened.

• For a protein-rich treat, top Greek yogurt with berries, almonds, and honey before freezing until hard.

• Dip apples, bananas, or strawberries in melted dark chocolate and put on parchment paper for a delectable, antioxidant-rich dessert.

Hydration And Beverage Options On A Flexitarian Diet

Proper hydration is critical for general health and well-being, and beverage selection may have a substantial influence on the nutritional profile of a flexitarian diet. Choosing hydrating and nutrient-dense beverages can help supplement meal options while also meeting hydration needs. Considerations include:

• To add taste and moisture to simple water, add slices of citrus fruits, cucumber, mint, or berries. Avoid adding sweets or artificial substances.

• Enjoy herbal teas like chamomile, peppermint, or ginger for hydration and possible health advantages including digestion and relaxation.

• Make smoothie bowls more nutritious by adding fruits, nuts, seeds, and granola for extra texture, taste, and moisture.

Maintaining a flexitarian diet while managing social settings and eating out takes adaptability and attentiveness. Planning, expressing preferences, and making educated choices allow you to enjoy social events and restaurant meals while adhering to flexitarian ideals. Strategies include:

• Communicate dietary preferences and limitations ahead of time to ensure appropriate alternatives are available.

• Consider menu modifications to accommodate a flexitarian diet, such as substituting plant-based proteins or adding more vegetables.

• Flexibility: Embrace flexibility and moderation when presented with restricted alternatives, concentrating on enjoying the social part of meals rather than rigid adherence to dietary standards.

CHAPTER FIVE

Flexitarian Diet For Weight Management

The flexitarian diet's focus on plant-based meals, lean meats, and whole grains might help weight control objectives by encouraging satiety, lowering calorie consumption, and delivering important nutrients. Strategies for weight control under a flexitarian paradigm include:

• Mindful eating and portion management may prevent overconsumption of calorie-dense foods, especially during meals with meat or high-fat alternatives.

• Prioritize plant-based foods, including fruits, vegetables, legumes, and whole grains, to enhance fullness and enjoyment.

• Combine a flexitarian diet with regular physical activity to achieve weight management objectives.

Include cardiovascular, strength, and flexibility exercises for total health and fitness.

Flexitarian Diet For Heart Health

The flexitarian diet's focus on plant-based foods and lean meats is consistent with dietary patterns linked with a lower risk of heart disease. The flexitarian diet may improve cardiovascular health by focusing on heart-healthy fats, fiber, and antioxidants. Key tactics include:

• Incorporate unsaturated fats like nuts, seeds, avocados, and olive oil to decrease cholesterol and lessen the risk of heart disease.

• Fiber-Rich Foods: Whole grains, fruits, vegetables, and legumes are excellent sources of dietary fiber, which helps decrease blood pressure, improve cholesterol levels, and promote heart health.

• Limit processed foods that have added sugars, bad fats, and salt, since these may lead to inflammation, high blood pressure, and other heart disease risks.

A Flexible Diet For Diabetes Management

The flexitarian diet, which emphasizes plant-based meals, lean proteins, and complex carbs, may help with blood sugar control and overall diabetes treatment. Individuals with diabetes may benefit from a flexitarian diet by concentrating on nutrient-dense, low-glycemic foods and eating in moderation. Strategies include:

• Choose complete, minimally processed carbs like fruits, vegetables, legumes, and whole grains to acquire key nutrients and fiber without causing blood sugar spikes.

• Monitor carbohydrate portion amounts to maintain blood sugar levels. Pair with lean meats and healthy fats for delayed digestion and satiety.

• Regularly monitor blood sugar levels and change food choices depending on individual reactions. Collaborate with healthcare specialists for optimal diabetes control.

Finally, adopting a flexitarian diet fosters health, environmental sustainability, and culinary innovation. Individuals may reap the advantages of a flexitarian lifestyle by integrating nutrient-dense snacks and appetizers, embracing hydration and beverage options, managing social settings and eating out, and adapting dietary choices to particular health objectives.

Flexitarian Diet For Digestive Health

The Flexitarian Diet encourages the consumption of fiber-rich plant foods such as fruits, vegetables, whole grains, legumes, and nuts. These foods improve digestive health by promoting regular bowel movements, preserving gut microbial diversity, and lowering the risk of gastrointestinal illnesses including constipation, diverticulosis, and colorectal cancer. Furthermore, the flexitarian diet's reduced consumption of processed foods and red meat promotes digestive health.

Flexitarian Diet For Healthy Aging

A flexitarian diet high in fruits, vegetables, and plant-based proteins contains vital minerals, antioxidants, and phytochemicals that promote healthy aging and lifespan.

These nutrients battle oxidative stress, inflammation, and cellular damage caused by aging, lowering the risk of age-related disorders including cardiovascular disease, cognitive decline, and some malignancies. The modest incorporation of lean meats and fish offers enough intake of protein and critical elements needed to preserve muscle strength and bone health as people age.

Flexitarian Diet For Athletic Performance

The Flexitarian Diet provides the ideal combination of carbs, proteins, and lipids for athletic performance and muscle rehabilitation. Plant-based carbs provide continuous energy release, and plant-based proteins include important amino acids required for muscle repair and development.

Consuming a range of colored fruits and vegetables also delivers antioxidants, which help minimize exercise-induced inflammation and oxidative stress, improving overall athletic performance and recovery.

Flexitarian Diet For Mental Wellbeing

The Flexitarian Diet has an abundance of nutrient-dense foods, especially those high in omega-3 fatty acids, vitamins, and minerals, which promote cognitive performance and mental well-being. According to studies, eating fruits, vegetables, healthy grains, nuts, and seeds lowers the risk of depression, anxiety, and cognitive impairment. Additionally, consuming fish and shellfish in moderation delivers omega-3 fatty acids, which are necessary for brain function and mood stability.

Flexitarian Diet for Environmental Sustainability: One of the most significant advantages of the Flexitarian Diet is its favorable influence on the environment. Individuals who choose plant-based diets over animal products may dramatically lower their carbon footprint, water consumption, and land use related to food production.

Plant-based diets consume fewer natural resources and emit fewer greenhouse gases than diets heavy on animal products. Adopting a flexitarian lifestyle may help to reduce climate change and preserve natural habitats for future generations.

CHAPTER SIX

Flexitarian Diet For Ethical Concerns

The Flexitarian Diet supports ethical issues by encouraging conscientious and sustainable eating choices. Individuals may help animals by lowering their intake of animal products and focusing on plant-based diets.

Choosing locally sourced, organic, and ethically produced foods improves the ethical integrity of the flexitarian lifestyle by ensuring that food production techniques are consistent with personal ideals of compassion and sustainability.

Flexitarian Diet For Families And Children

The Flexitarian Diet is a family-friendly approach to healthy eating, with flexibility and adaptation to fit different tastes and nutritional demands within the home. Parents may develop good eating habits and encourage lifetime healthiness in their children by exposing them to a variety of plant-based meals from a young age. Involving children in meal planning and preparation may help them develop a good connection with food and adopt experimental eating habits.

Flexitarian Diet on a Budget: Despite popular belief, healthy eating does not have to be costly. Plant-based staples including beans, lentils, nutritious grains, and seasonal veggies are frequently less expensive than meat or processed diets. Meal planning, bulk shopping, and reducing food waste may all help you save money on groceries while increasing nutritional value.

Furthermore, growing herbs, fruits, and vegetables at home or engaging in community-supported agriculture (CSA) programs may be inexpensive ways to include fresh, locally produced products into a flexitarian diet.

A flexitarian diet might be difficult to follow when traveling, but it is not impossible. Here are some tips:

1. Pack Snacks: Nuts, seeds, dried fruits, and whole grain crackers provide fast and healthy snacks on the move.

2. Explore Local Cuisine: Learn about the local food culture and search for flexitarian-friendly alternatives including salads, vegetable-based dishes, and tofu or legume-based meals.

3. Choose Flexitarian-Friendly Restaurants: Look for restaurants that provide a choice of plant-based alternatives alongside animal dishes, enabling you to tailor your meal to your flexitarian needs.

4. Choose Flexitarian Fast Food: Many fast-food restaurants now offer plant-based alternatives such

as veggie burgers or salads, making it simpler to maintain your flexitarian diet while on the go.

Flexitarian Diet For Special Events & Holidays

Keeping a flexitarian diet for special events and holidays may be pleasurable with the following suggestions:

1. Plan Ahead: If you're attending a party or function, volunteer to bring a flexitarian-friendly meal to guarantee there's something for you to eat.

2. Focus on Vegetables: Make colorful vegetables, salads, and vegetable-based meals the major components of your meal.

3. Be Mindful of quantities: If meat or animal products are provided, eat fewer quantities and balance them out with bigger servings of plant-based options.

4. Experiment with Plant-Based foods: Use special occasions to attempt new and intriguing plant-based foods that will appeal to both flexitarians and non-flexitarians.

Flexitarian Diet For Busy Lifestyles

For individuals with hectic schedules, the flexitarian diet provides flexibility and convenience:

1. Meal Prep: Set aside some time each week for meal preparation, concentrating on batch-cooking plant-based staples such as grains, legumes, and roasted vegetables that can be easily integrated into meals throughout the week.

2. rapid and Easy Meals: Keep basic and healthy flexitarian-friendly foods on hand, such as canned beans, pre-washed greens, and frozen veggies, for rapid meal prep.

3. Utilize Convenience Foods: When cooking from scratch is not possible, use convenience foods such

as pre-packaged salads, frozen veggie burgers, and canned soups that fall within the flexitarian framework.

4. One-pot dishes: For a healthy and convenient supper alternative, choose one-pot dishes that mix protein-rich beans or tofu with a variety of veggies and grains.

A Flexitarian Diet For Pregnancy And Breastfeeding

While following a flexitarian diet, it is essential to guarantee appropriate nutrition throughout pregnancy and lactation.

1. Focus on Nutrient-Dense Foods: To satisfy higher nutritional demands, eat more fruits and vegetables, whole grains, legumes, nuts, seeds, and fortified plant-based milk substitutes.

2. Consult a Healthcare Professional: Collaborate with a healthcare physician or registered dietitian to

create a food plan that accommodates both your flexitarian choices and nutritional needs while pregnant and nursing.

3. Monitor Iron Intake: Include iron-rich plant foods like as lentils, tofu, spinach, and fortified cereals in your diet, and if necessary, take a prenatal vitamin containing iron.

4. Stay Hydrated: Stay hydrated by drinking lots of water and other fluids throughout the day, particularly if you are nursing.

Flexitarian Diet For Menopause

Flexitarian diets may improve general health and well-being throughout menopause.

1. Focus on Plant-Based Phytoestrogens: Include foods high in phytoestrogens, such as soy products (tofu, tempeh, edamame), flaxseeds, sesame seeds, and whole grains, which may help ease menopausal symptoms.

2. Include Calcium-Rich Foods: To maintain bone health, eat calcium-rich plant foods such as leafy greens, almonds, fortified plant-based milk, and calcium-set tofu.

3. Prioritize Omega-3 Fatty Acids: To improve heart health and decrease inflammation, eat omega-3 fatty acids from sources such as walnuts, chia seeds, flaxseeds, and hemp seeds.

4. Moderate Caffeine and Alcohol Consumption: Limit your caffeine and alcohol intake since they might increase menopausal symptoms like hot flashes and alter sleep patterns.

Flexitarian Diet For Longevity

The flexitarian diet may help to lifespan and general health by encouraging a balanced consumption of plant-based foods.

1. Emphasize Whole Foods: Build your diet around whole, minimally processed plant foods like fruits,

vegetables, whole grains, legumes, nuts, and seeds, which are high in vitamins, minerals, fiber, and antioxidants.

2. Limit Processed Foods: Consume less processed and ultra-processed foods rich in added sugars, bad fats, and salt, which have been related to chronic illnesses and premature aging.

3. Include a range of plant-based protein sources, such as beans, lentils, chickpeas, tofu, tempeh, nuts, and seeds, to ensure that you get enough protein for muscle maintenance and repair.

4. Stay Active: Combine a flexitarian diet with regular physical exercise to improve overall health, manage weight, and lower your risk of age-related chronic illnesses.

CHAPTER SEVEN

Flexitarian Diet with Food Allergies Or Intolerances

For those with dietary allergies or intolerances, the flexitarian diet provides flexibility and options:

1. Emphasize full, unprocessed plant foods to reduce allergy exposure and maintain a balanced diet.

2. Read Labels Carefully: Before buying packaged or processed goods, carefully read the ingredient labels to avoid any allergies or intolerances.

3. Experiment with substitutes: Look into alternate ingredients and substitutes to meet particular dietary requirements, such as utilizing plant-based milk alternatives instead of dairy, or tofu or tempeh instead of meat.

4. Consult a Healthcare Professional: Collaborate with a healthcare professional or qualified dietitian

to create a meal plan that satisfies your nutritional requirements while avoiding allergies and intolerances.

Flexitarian Diet And Food Sensitivities

For those with food sensitivities, the flexitarian diet offers a flexible approach to addressing dietary restrictions:

1. Identify Trigger Foods: Maintain a food diary to identify possible trigger foods and follow symptoms to better understand your specific food sensitivities.

2. Focus on Diversity: Include a broad range of plant-based meals to guarantee a diversified nutritional intake and limit the risk of developing sensitivities to certain substances.

3. Cook from Scratch: Make meals from scratch with fresh, whole foods to get more control over what

goes into your diet and avoid hidden causes of sensitivity.

4. Consider an Elimination Diet: If required, follow an elimination diet with the help of a healthcare expert to identify particular trigger foods and assess your unique sensitivities.

Flexitarian Diet To Manage Chronic Conditions

The flexitarian diet may help manage chronic illnesses by encouraging a nutrient-dense, plant-based eating pattern:

1. Anti-Inflammatory Foods: To help decrease inflammation caused by chronic illnesses, eat foods high in antioxidants, omega-3 fatty acids, and fiber, such as fruits, vegetables, whole grains, nuts, seeds, and fatty fish.

2. Limit Added Sugars and Saturated Fats: Limit your consumption of added sugars, refined carbs,

and saturated fats found in processed and fried foods, which may aggravate the symptoms of chronic illnesses including diabetes, cardiovascular disease, and arthritis.

3. Limit your sodium consumption by eating whole, minimally processed foods and flavoring meals with herbs, spices, and lemon juice instead of salt, which may help control illnesses such as hypertension and heart disease.

4. Stay Consistent: Eat a well-balanced diet rich in nutrient-dense plant foods to promote overall health and manage symptoms of chronic diseases over time.

Conclusion

The flexitarian diet provides a flexible and inclusive approach to nutrition that may be tailored to a variety of lifestyles, dietary choices, and health requirements. Whether you're traveling, celebrating a special occasion, managing a busy schedule, navigating pregnancy or menopause, aiming for longevity, dealing with food allergies or sensitivities, or managing chronic conditions, the flexitarian diet offers practical strategies and guidelines for incorporating more plant-based foods into your meals while still allowing for the occasional consumption of animal products.

Individuals may obtain the health advantages of a flexitarian diet by choosing whole, minimally processed plant foods and adopting a broad and balanced eating pattern.

www.ingramcontent.com/pod-product-compliance
Lightning Source LLC
Chambersburg PA
CBHW051910250726
48659CB00002B/575